Lose Weight, Stop Stress and Make Better Love

5 Easy Steps
by Training Your Brain

to Phyllis,

With every good wish
a appreciation.

Frank Sommer.

Mobile App

Apple Store:
Stress Relief by Dr. Frank

Google Play – Android mobiles:
5 Easy Steps to Stress Relief

Dr. Frank G. Sommers is a psychiatrist, author, and filmmaker. A former member of the Faculty of Medicine, University of Toronto, and of the Canadian Forces (Reserves) with service in Afghanistan, he is in private practice of couple and sexual therapy in Toronto.

Praise for

Lose Weight, Stop Stress and Make Better Love

———•✦•———

The reason you should take the time to read this booklet by Dr. Sommers is because it works. I am a patient of Dr. Sommers. I have applied his techniques and guides for stress management and weight loss.

Most of us are under stress or will be at some point in our lives and most of us are aware, that when we are under stress, one of the things we do for comfort, or lack of time is eating the wrong foods at the wrong times.

Dr. Sommers' booklet is succinct, to the point, and easy to follow. The easy part will be reading it. The more challenging part will be applying it. You will have to want to make the change, and be disciplined about doing the relaxation exercises and eating the right foods which offer the most nutrition for your body.

As with all worthwhile programs nothing in life comes for free except Love. You will have to wait to start to see and feel the results, so stick with it and follow the 5 steps and watch your life change for the better, forever. IT WORKS!

You will find a lot of information out there in book stores and magazine subscriptions. If you are a nutritionist, researcher, or just love to read, by all means read the books, magazines and internet blogs. With this booklet you can read it in an hour and get started right away.

Here is to your happy present centred, and process absorbed new you.

P.N.

───·•·───

One of the most useful things about the "soldier's (KAF*) card" has been the way it not only calms me, but quickly helps me return to thinking clearly (even if only in part)! My wife and I have regularly stressful interactions with each other, as well as with my mother, our friends, co-workers, even our doctors. We do not always follow all five steps while under pressure (we forget), but we always solve problems easier when we do remember the steps! I personally find the sensory check and positive self-talk are the most helpful of these. Once we can think again, we make a better team again.

S.K.

*KAF stands for Kandahar Air Field in Afghanistan, where Dr. Sommers served as the psychiatrist, and taught his 5 Step Method of Stress Relief to soldiers.

───·•·───

I have always been very sceptical, never fully allowing myself to engage in any techniques or self-help methods that were aimed towards dealing with stress relief. Unfortunately I relied greatly on anxiety medications, or many times alcohol as my coping mechanism to mask/deal with the everyday stresses in life. As with the KAF* (wallet) card I also reluctantly began to experiment and implement the techniques taught to me. Much to my surprise I was, and to this day am, overwhelmed by the impact this simple method has had on my life. My KAF card is to me part of my every day routine as I would breathe, eat and sleep. As if it were second nature, not a day that goes by that I do not utilise my KAF* card. I have such a great peace of mind that now without the use of any medications I can control my reactions when faced with everyday decisions that otherwise would have consumed my every thought with the "what if's" and "what would have's" that have kept me from moving forward in many areas of my life. I would strongly urge anyone sceptical or not, be open minded and have faith in this technique, as it truly will change your life. It did mine.

A.R.

————•—•————

Firstly I'd just like to say a few things about Dr. Sommers.

I came into this program thinking it would help me with my sexual health. I have learned SO MUCH more than that. It's been about life lessons and about love. Although our work isn't done yet – I'm extremely appreciative of everything he has helped teach me thus far.

In terms of the KAF 5 steps – I'd like to call out a few of the steps that have been extremely helpful with my development.

Using the 5 senses is one of the best exercises on many levels. It makes you stop thinking about the next thing or the last thing – you can't help but think about the only thing that matters which is the present. It's helped me heighten my senses which helps to give me appreciation, amongst other things.

The tandem of thought stopping and positive self talk have also been invaluable. My favourite quote is "the world is a mirror of your own beliefs". My world (your world) can get better if you simply focus on not going into the dark alleys of life and rather build up your confidence by thinking about why you're prepared to be great. These are not just sexual health tools – they are also life tools, and I'm glad they're becoming a key part of my tool kit. Thanks Dr. Sommers.

M.B.

Professional Endorsements

"A clinically sophisticated approach to weight management that provides down to earth guidance for working with stress and other triggers of emotional eating."

Dr. Zindel B. Segal, Ph.D., C.Psych.
Cameron Wilson Chair in Depression Studies
Professor of Psychiatry
University of Toronto

———•+•———

"This is an insightful, practical book and an easy read to achieve most in life we truly want. It is from a master psychiatric clinician and researcher of sexuality and stress reduction. It's easy to accomplish the simple 5 steps to avoid and reduce anxiety and stress. To do it inspires and satisfies. It works. Eat and love better. Everyone begin now."

Dr. Gordon D. Jensen, M.D.
Life Fellow, American Psychiatric Association
Emeritus Professor of Psychiatry
University of California, School of Medicine, Davis

———•+•———

"This looks interesting. It incorporates elements of CBT, Mindfulness and relaxation therapy. It will be very helpful."

Dr. Valerie H. Taylor, MD, PhD, FRCPC
Psychiatrist-in-chief, Women's College Hospital
Associate Professor, University of Toronto
Mental Health Chair, Canadian Obesity Network

———•◆•———

"I think this book is so practical and down to earth that everyone should read it. It makes so much sense that everyone can benefit."

Dr. Peggy J. Kleinplatz, Ph.D.
Professor, Faculty of Medicine
Clinical Professor, School of Psychology
University of Ottawa

———•◆•———

Frank G. Sommers, MD

"It's not stress that kills us, it is our reaction to it"

"Every stress leaves an indelible scar, and the organism pays for its survival after a stressful situation by becoming a little older."

Hans Selye, MD
Father of Stress Science
(1907 – 1982)

Lose Weight, Stop Stress and Make Better Love

5 Easy Steps by Training Your Brain

Frank G. Sommers, MD

Fellow, Royal College of Physicians of Canada
Distinguished Fellow, American Psychiatric Association

Health, Wellness, Nutrition & Sexuality

A Pathway Health Book

Note: The information contained in this book is not intended to substitute
for professional or medical advice. The author and Pathway Productions
Inc. disclaim responsibility or liability for any loss that maybe incurred as a
result of the use or application of any information included herein.
Readers should always consult their physician or other professional for
treatment or advice.

Library and Archives Canada Cataloguing in Publication

Sommers, Frank G

Lose Weight, Stop Stress and Make Better Love / Frank G. Sommers.

Includes bibliographical references.
ISBN 978-0-9877800-1-0
1. Stress management. 2. Weight loss. 3. Sex instruction. I. Title.

BF575.S75S67 2012   158.1   C2012-902950-5

For additional, helpful materials please visit website:
stressrelief.drsommers.com

Visit Mobile App

Apple Store:
Stress Relief by Dr. Frank

Google Play – Android mobiles:
5 Easy Steps to Stress Relief

For Eva, Robert and Daniel
and all our Family, current and future.

Towards a world with less anxiety and strife,
where people everywhere realize
what we have in common
is much greater than what divides us.

Frank Sommers, MD, FRCPC, DFAPA

Contents

Praise for 3

Professional Endorsements 7

5 Easy Steps To Stress Relief. 19

We know there is a better way. 19

Stress Immunization With Brain Power
      and Your Autonomic Nervous System . 21

The Two Basic Principles:
      Present Centred (P.C.) and
      Process Absorbed (P.A.) 24

Weight Management. 39

Obesity and Overweight 39

Make Better Love. 51

Appendix 1: Stress Immunization Wallet Card 61

Appendix 2: Relaxation Images 63

Appendix 3: Personal Daily Weight Control Log 69

Dear Reader,

Here you will find the path to tranquility in your busy, at times turbulent, life. '**Lose Weight, Stop Stress and Make Better Love in 5 Easy Steps By Training Your Brain**' is a clinically and battlefield-tested way to calm your inner turmoil without drugs, no matter what may be happening in your life and around you. Using the power of your brain and nervous system, you will reinforce your inner strength to deal with adversity, and achieve inner peace and harmony.

Further, use this brief, very effective guide to help you conquer overeating, and thus fight weight-gain and obesity. This is now becoming a major health issue in many peoples' lives.

Lose Weight, Stop Stress and Make Better Love in 5 Easy Steps By Training Your Brain takes a very different approach to the problem of weight gain. Once again, using our brain power and built-in nervous system we can modify, if not eliminate, a major cause of unhealthy eating: stress.

Reach your potential, and conquer your stress reaction. You owe it to yourself to try it.

Furthermore, as you modify your nervous system's response to stress you will find (as do my patients) a major enhancement, and intensity in your love making. Thus, here is one more reason for you to embark on this exciting journey using the knowledge you will gain from my little book.

Sincerely,

Dr. Frank G. Sommers, MD, FRCPC

Frank G. Sommers, MD

PART I

5 Easy Steps
To Stress Relief

The tools and concepts I'm sharing with you in this little guide can change your life.

Life is stressful. Alcohol and drugs, and yes, food, are ways to try to handle stress. But though they may provide momentary relief, ultimately they're not the solution.

We know there is a better way.

Modern brain research has established that we can train our brain, and nervous system to make us more resilient. The techniques you'll learn here arise from many years of my work as a clinical psychiatrist delivering care to thousands of men and women, singles and couples, children and families.

My aim here is not to bury you in heavy reading of myriad facts, stories, or research, and thereby add to the stress you are trying to conquer. Time is short and life is precious. And, let's face it, many people don't like to read. So, in this little guide I'm going to give you the very practical steps that you can start using today to become a more balanced, happier person.

While I have been teaching my patients and students over many years the steps of my program, it really all came together in its current form during my work in Afghanistan with the deployed military.

In that war zone, one of the most common problems I had to treat was acute anxiety, or stress, particularly in soldiers who were being sent on dangerous missions out from the relative safety of our base. This is called going 'outside the wire'. Some of these soldiers experienced difficulty sleeping or eating. They often felt tired, listless, depressed.

But all felt very anxious.

While there is a whole bunch of pills I could have given out to help them cope, I wanted to find a better way, without drugs, to help the soldiers. This way they would be free of medication side effects, and remain more alert and able to function effectively as part of their team.

I call my program:

Frank G. Sommers, MD

Stress Immunization With Brain Power and Your Autonomic Nervous System

I'll explain shortly what this all means. I'm glad to say that the soldiers were very receptive to the **5 Steps** in this short program, and coming back from missions they told me how useful they found it.

Upon returning from Afghanistan, I consolidated and further refined my program. The ongoing feedback from my patients has also been very positive.

A Brief Note on our Nervous System

The brain sends signals to all parts of the body via the Central Nervous System (CNS) travelling through or adjacent to the spinal cord.

A part of this very efficient network is the Autonomic Nervous System (ANS). Its two sub-components, called the Sympathetic and the Parasympathetic systems are of great importance in dealing with stress.

The Sympathetic is the alarm or 'fight or flight' system, efficiently responding to stress from any source. On the other hand, when the Parasympathetic system is engaged we feel relaxed and calm. Through the Principle of Reciprocal Inhibition, both systems can't be "on", as it were, at the same time.

A note on my 'Prescription' for Stress Immunization

You'll see that there are two formats of the prescription. The large one (Figure 1) is easily visualized and helps initial learning. The small version you'll find in Appendix 1 as Figure 2. I suggest you laminate and place this one in your wallet for ever-ready availability, application and practise. Soldiers told me that they kept the small one in their front packet, as a 'soldier's card' – enabling them to readily review the **5 Steps**, even during a lull in fighting. Frequent review is a good idea, and I encourage all my patients (and family) to do the same. Repeated reviews of the **5 Steps** will help to fix them in your mind, and practising them will promote or facilitate your nervous system re-training, or programming. This is the essential core or backbone of my approach.

You can also download the 5 Steps to Stress Relief in a smart phone app available from the Apple store **(Stress Relief by Dr. Frank)** and the Android Mobiles **(5 Easy Steps to Stress Relief)**. Many people are finding this app with the reminder feature, calming music and relaxing pictures very helpful.

So, here is my prescription:

As you can see (Figure 1) there are **5 Steps** that make up my 'prescription'. But before I explain each step, let me make clear what this important diagram and the letters P.C./P.A. mean. They are life changing.

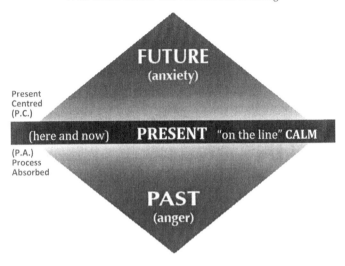

STRESS IMMUNIZATION
With Brain Power and Autonomic Training

FUTURE
(anxiety)

Present
Centred
(P.C.)

(here and now) **PRESENT** "on the line" **CALM**

(P.A.)
Process
Absorbed

PAST
(anger)

HOW TO GET ON THE LINE
Step1: 5 Sense check list (see, hear, touch, taste, smell)
Step 2: Deep abdominal breathing 3 times a day
Step 3: Thought stopping
Step 4: Positive self talk
Step 5: Images/Pictures that soothe you *PLUS relaxation*

PRACTISE THESE 5 STEPS OFTEN

© Frank Sommers, MD, FRCPC, ROLE 3 MMU, KAF, Dec 07, Afghanistan

Figure 1

The Two Basic Principles: P.C. and P.A.
(Present Centred and Process Absorbed)

Most people would agree that life happens in the present, the 'here and now'.

These two Principles, which I've been teaching for over 35 years, deal with the passage of time.

The First Principle

This is the ability to be **Present Centred** (P.C. for short). This means that in your mind you are not thinking about the future or the past. The Future is what may happen the next second, minute, hour, day, or a million years from now, and everything in between. And the Past is what happened a second or a million years ago, and everything in between. The straight line in the diagram represents the 'flow' of the Present. In reality, this is where life happens. Right here, right now.

The Future

Let's agree that anytime you're thinking about anything in the future, you're above the line. This is where anxiety resides, which is really the fear of something painful happening in the future. This is where you're thinking about what will be, what could be, what might be, what won't be, why it won't be, and so on.

Frank G. Sommers, MD

The Past

Let's further agree that whenever you're think-ing about anything in the past, you're below the line. This is where you're thinking what was, what wasn't, could have been, etc. As I tell my patients, in both of these cases it's as if you're spinning the wheels of your car in a snowbank. You're stuck, not moving anywhere. A predominant negative emo-tion residing here often is anger, guilt, or regret.

The Present

To be able to be 'on the line', or totally in the Present, that is to be 'Present Centred' (P.C.), enables you to be Calm. It's an energized state where you feel more 'alive'. Here you're better able to work, love, and laugh, in a comfortable, confident manner, able to engage with others. It is 'life affirming'.

The Second Principle

This is related to the First. I call it being '**Process Absorbed**' (P.A. for short). I define this state as the opposite of being 'goal-directed'. Much of life is goal-directed, and some people even make 'to do' lists, which can, for some, become a ritual obses-sion. While goals, properly utilized, can aid accomplishment, our ability to engage in the flow of a task, or in love making, for example, is enhanced if we understand how this Second Principle can enrich our lives. An example can illuminate this. Imagine seeing little children playing on a sandy beach, build-ing sandcastles, or in a wading pool on a hot summer day. The children are totally caught up in what they are doing, and enjoying every moment. They're not distracted by irrelevant thoughts, such as what they had for breakfast, or what they'll do in the evening. They're enjoying the moment-to-moment activity that they are doing. They are caught up in the experience of what they're doing at that moment. In other words, they are Process Absorbed (P.A.).

These *2 Principles* have formed an essential core of my therapy with patients who are suffering from a range of difficulties in their personal, intimate lives.

So, understanding these *2 Principles* is quite important. But the question arises: how do we get 'On The Line' where we feel Calm? How do we not think, or fret, or worry about the future, or ruminate on the past? This is where brain training comes in, fortunately in a very effective way.

Let's look at it this way.

We human beings have basically four ways of interacting with the world around us. Thinking is one way. This takes place in the 'newer' brain, the so-called neocortex. Feeling is a second way, which happens in the older part of the brain, the archicortex, or limbic lobe. Intuition is a third way, probably the result of super-fast thinking and feeling.

But the fourth way, often neglected, is our sensory brain in yet another brain location, dealing with our *5 Senses*.

This fourth way is very important for us because using our 5 Senses in a very deliberate way enables us to climb onto the centre line, and become **Present Centred** and **Process Absorbed**, and Calm.

So here are my **5 Steps**:

Step 1: The Crucial Role of Sensing

Fortunately, we can all learn to become more mindful of our senses. To this end I ask all my patients to do a sensory checklist three to five times a day. I suggest you too try this exercise. Simply stop whatever you are doing for a moment, and ask yourself "What am I sensing now?" i.e. what do I 'see, hear, touch, taste and smell'. This sensory checklist only takes a few seconds, and helps to center or ground you totally in the present ('on the line') in a very concrete way. In effect, it resets our brain circuitry. And remember, when you're 'on the line' you can't be anxious. Practising this regularly will help you to relieve stress, fear, and anxiety.

Note: In doing the sensing exercise you may well find that a sense organ is not engaged at that moment. For example you're not tasting, or smelling anything at the moment you do your sensory check. Your answer 'nothing' then is quite O.K. The important point is that by asking the question you have helped to re-focus your brain's activity.

Sensing – some further words

By sensing I mean paying close attention (or being mindful) to the moment-to-moment information we perceive through our 5 Senses: what we see, hear, touch, taste and smell. Our senses are always working (if we're healthy), bringing to our brain a variety of stimuli, or information. However, often we remain unaware of this information unless it happens to be out of the ordinary. For example, when you hear a siren going by your window your ears pick it up, and your brain's auditory attention focuses on it. Once it recedes, your senses will focus on some other item, event, or stimulus that will engage your attention such as the curtain moving when a strong gust of wind blows through an open window, or your nose picks up a sweet scent walking past a bakery.

As we focus consciously, with heightened awareness on our senses, we are able to become **Present Centred** and fully *mindful* of the moment. We are 'on the line', and in truth, this is where life happens. All thoughts (a different part of our brain) of the future, eg. what will be, could be, might be, etc; or thoughts of the past, eg. what was, wasn't, could have been, etc. are really 'figments of our imagination' so to speak. In our model (see Figure 1), we're above the line when thinking about the Future, or below the line when thinking about the Past.

By doing our 5 Sense check, we are able to focus our brain on the present moment. We are re-setting our internal rheostat, as it were. Importantly, you are liberating yourself from worries about the future, remembering that anxiety is expectation of pain in the future, and liberating yourself from pre-occupying or lingering emotions from the past, such as anger.

By being 'on the line' you achieve a state of feeling energized calm, and relaxed. With practise this can help to lower blood pressure, and improve the immune system and our overall health.

In time, this can become our pathway to serenity.

Now let's consider other important elements of the 'prescription':

Step 2: Breathing (Deeply)

We tend to be shallow breathers most of the time, and in conditions of anxiety often hold our breath. In fact, next time you notice you're holding your breath, ask yourself if you could be anxious. Frequently the answer will be yes. One or two slow, deep abdominal breaths will be very helpful to relieve this state.

I recommend linking deep breathing exercises to the sensing checklist done three or four times a day. Most people find this so helpful that its use for stress relief becomes second nature. Remember that deep abdominal breathing means your abdomen expands fully as you breathe in, and contracts fully on breathing out. Try this right now.

Step 3: Thought Stopping

To understand this important tool in brain training let's go back to the soldiers in Afghanistan.

Let's say one day Corporal Jones gets tasked, together with his small team, to leave the relative security of our main base the next day, and drive 'outside the wire', to resupply fellow soldiers stationed at an FOB (Forward Operating Base), bringing them food, water, mail, etc. This can actually be a rather dangerous task. Often there is only one possible road to the FOB and attacks on the road can and do occur frequently. Corporal Jones can recall that just the other week on a similar assignment, one of his good buddies got his legs blown off when an IED (Improvised Explosive Device) hit their vehicle.

On another occasion, a few weeks earlier, another IED blast claimed the lives of three members of another team.

We need to recognize and accept that our thoughts have consequences, sometimes very undesirable, negative ones, including feelings of anxiety, despair, hopelessness and depression, as well as anger and rage. Thoughts like these can be very heavy on the psyche, impairing one's ability to feel, and function "as normal".

Stopping these negative thoughts (I call them 'Dark Alleys') from occupying your brain is possible, important, and beneficial. The method seems simple, but can be highly effective as *part* of the overall program of Stress Immunization. You say to yourself: "Stop, I am not going there." This is an effective self-instruction to your brain to stop or cease this unproductive, possibly harmful thought.

To further explain this, I tell my patients to imagine they're walking down a well-lit street late at night, when they come up to a Dark Alley which would be a shortcut to their destination. Would you take it? Most people would not. They would keep going on the well-lit road, longer but safer. Our mind throws up all kinds of 'Dark Alleys' and we need to develop the mental discipline to not go there, or yield to them. The reality is that any of us could become overwhelmed, anxious or depressed if we allowed ourselves to enter these 'Dark Alleys'. The good news is to recognize that we have some control and to learn to apply it.

It is vital for Corporal Jones to stop his negative thoughts/ memories of the painful tragedies in the past, and channel his *brain power* in a way that promotes his ability to function well in the present. Thought Stopping is an important tool for this.

Note: The action I advise here does *not* imply that we never think about the future or the past. But it means that we do it with awareness of the present. In other words, you would 'say' to yourself "**now** I am considering, or planning the future, or **now** I am reflecting on the past." This way you retain control of your thought processes and moderate potential negative emotions.

Step 4: Positive Self-Talk

This is also an important and effective skill to become familiar with, and to master, on the way to coping successfully or adaptively with stress. In my experience, not many people are really good at this.

Thinking back to Corporal Jones' dangerous assignment, what would his positive self-talk be? Would you agree this is a good example, "I'm a lucky guy. Nothing's ever happened to me. I'll be all right."

Well, if you think that, you wouldn't be right. Positive Self-Talk needs to be *grounded in reality*. In this example Corporal Jones' helpful, confidence-boosting script would be, "I'm competent, capable, and well-trained, with a good team. I have faith I can get through this."

Please note and recall the difference. This kind of Positive Self-Talk is especially important when you are facing a fearful situation, or you're actually in a situation of heightened danger or anxiety.

Our brain is a wonderful organ, capable of rapid response to stimuli. Our self-caring task is to provide it, or program it, with those stimuli which will help us to get through sticky, anxiety-provoking situations.

This would apply not just to soldiers in a war zone, but to people in all sorts of situations. The more adept you become at developing *appropriate* self-talk, the more effectively you will be able to lower your stress level, and thus cope with a task, challenge, or situation. It is vital that you are able to do this quickly when the chips are down, in an emergency.

Once you try this a few times you will notice that Positive Self-Talk can replicate the support, or equal the boost in confidence you would get from an outside source that you trust and whose experience and expertise you respect. This in turn enables you to settle down and apply all your knowledge, skill, and experience to the matter at hand, with focused attention, undiluted by fearful, self-defeating negative self-talk.

Step 5: Soothing/Relaxing Imagery

Another important attribute of the human brain probably unique to our species is our ability to imagine.

An interesting experiment that somewhat illuminates this is where people just watching a fireplace on a TV screen felt warm in their finger tips. I think just imagining a fireplace could achieve the same effect, at least in some people. Another example of the important contribution of imagery comes from the field of sex therapy where low-desire problems affect more and more men and women, especially in modern-day, stress-filled lives.

In the presence of normal hormone levels, and in the absence of illness, or severe marital or relationship discord, exercising one's erotic imagination can be a powerful aid in raising or reinforcing libido, or sexual appetite. Training ourselves to use the power of our imagination can yield very desirable benefits in many aspects of our lives.

For most people a nature scene can be very relaxing (see Appendix 2). Through our imagination we can recreate at least one nature scene where either we had or could have a pleasant experience. We can also use a photo, painting, or movie scene that brought a pleasurable feeling to us. By keeping one or two or three such scenes in our brain's '*imagination library*' we can practise going to this place in our mind's eye, and gain benefits similar to taking an actual journey there.

I think regular practise of this unique human ability trains your brain to send signals via your autonomic nervous system to the rest of your body. Through the activation of your parasympathetic system, you enjoy the benefits of relaxation.

And, remember, when you are relaxed, you can't be anxious.

Conclusion

It is important to realize that all stress or anxiety is channelled through the same parts of our nervous system. So regardless whether your stress is triggered by financial, work or employment issues, or family/relationship troubles, your stress response always involves similar nerve, endocrine, and brain structures. Fortunately, we can train the components of this system to moderate how we respond to stress.

So, there you have it: the *5 Steps of Stress Relief* which can enable you to modify or conquer your stress response to a manageable and productive level. This can lead to positive changes not only in your mental health and resiliency, but also impact on your vulnerability to many illnesses and ailments where stress plays a role.

And as you'll see in the following sections you will have the essential tools to achieve a healthier weight, and even enrich your love life.

In our increasingly globalized, 24/7 connected, stressful world, learning 'Stress First Aid' is an essential life skill. Make the effort to learn and put into practice this **5 Step** program, and see for yourself how your daily life becomes lighter, and happier, as your burdens lift, like gently floating red balloons, towards a clear blue sky.

The 5 Steps to Conquer Stress

■ Sensory Checklist (What do I See, Hear, Touch, Taste, Smell?)

■ Deep Abdominal Breathing

■ Thought Stopping

■ Positive Self-Talk

■ Soothing, Relaxing Imagery/Relaxation

Presentation of Dr. Frank Sommers *'Stress Immunization by Training Your Brain in 5 Easy Steps'* Program can be arranged. Please contact pathwayhealth@aol.com

Stress Studies

Adam TC, Epel ES. Stress, eating and the reward system. *Physiology & Behavior* (2007), 91(4):449-58.

Block JP, He Y, Ayanian JZ, et al. Psychosocial stress and change in weight among US adults. *American Journal of Epidemiology* (2009), 170(2): 181-192.

Daubenmier J, Lin J, Blackburn E, et al. Changes in stress, eating, and metabolic factors are related to changes in telomerase activity in randomized mindfulness intervention pilot study. *Psychoneuroendocrinology* (2011), Dec 12. [Epub ahead of print].

Daubenmier J, Kristeller J, Hecht FM, et al. Mindfulness Intervention for Stress Eating to Reduce Cortisol and Abdominal Fat among Overweight and Obese Women: An Exploratory Randomized Controlled Study. *Journal of Obesity* (2011), 2011:651936. Epub 2011 Oct 2.

Groesz LM, McCoy S, Carl J, et al. What is eating you? Stress and the drive to eat. *Appetite* (2012), 58(2):717-21.

Jastreboff AM, Potenza MN, Lacadie C, et al. Body mass index, metabolic factors, and striatal activation during stressful and neutral-relaxing states: an FMRI study. *Neuropsychopharmacology* (2011), 36(3):627-37.

Marchand WR. Mindfulness-based stress reduction, mindfulness-based cognitive therapy, and zen meditation for depression, anxiety, pain, and psychological distress. *Journal of Psychiatric Practice* (2012), 18(4):233-52.

Ornish D, Scherwitz LW, Billings JH, et al. Intensive Lifestyle Changes for Reversal of Coronary Heart Disease. *The Journal of American Medical Association* (1998), 280(23):2001-2007.

Peters A, Langemann D. Stress and eating behavior. *F1000 Biology Reports* (2010), 2:13.

Tomiyama AJ, Dallman MF, Epel ES. Comfort food is comforting to those most stressed: Evidence of the chronic stress response network in high stress women. *Psychoneuroendocrinology* (2011), 36(10): 1513-1519.

Torres SJ, Nowson CA. Relationship between stress, eating behaviour, and obesity. *Nutrition* (2007), 23(11-12):887-94.

Warne JP. Shaping the stress response: Interplay of palatable food choice, glucocotricoids insulin and abdominal obesity. *Molecular and Cellular Endocrinology* (2009), 300(1-2):137-46.

Workplace and Stress

Berset M, Semmer NK, Elfering A, et al. Does Stress at work make you gain weight? A two-year longitudinal study. *Scandinavian Journal of Work, Environment & Health* (2011), 37(1)45-53.

Nevanperä NJ, Hopsu L, Kuosma E, et al. Occupational burnout, eating behaviour, and weight among working women. *American Journal of Clinical Nutrition* (2012) Feb 29. [Epub ahead of print].

Nilsson PM, Klasson EB, Nyberg P. Life-style intervention at the worksite – reduction of cardiovascular risk factors in a randomized study. *Scandinavian Journal of Work, Environment & Health* (2001), 27(1):57-62.

Petterson IL, Arnetz BB. Psychosocial stressors and well-being in health care workers. The impact of an intervention program. *Social Science and Medicine* (1998), 47(11):1763-72.

Rahe RH, Taylor CB, Tolles RL, et al. A novel stress and coping workplace program reduces illness and healthcare utilization. *Psychosomatic Medicine* (2002), 64:278-286.

Interested employers please contact Pathway's '*Workplace Anti-Stress (WAS) Program*' at: pathwayhealth@aol.com

Resources

Apple Store:	Stress Relief by Dr. Frank
For Android Mobiles:	5 Easy Steps to Stress Relief
Visit on the Web:	Stressrelief.drsommers.com

The Mindful Way through Depression. Williams M, Teasdale J, Segal Z, Kabat-Zinn J. The Guilford Press, New York, 2007.

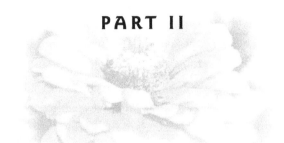

PART II

Weight Management

Obesity and Overweight

Key facts

- Worldwide obesity has more than doubled since 1980.

- In 2008, 1.5 billion adults, 20 and older, were overweight. Of these over 200 million men and nearly 300 million women were obese.

- 65% of the world's population live in countries where overweight and obesity kills more people than underweight.

- Nearly 43 million children under the age of five were overweight in 2010.

- Obesity is preventable.

World Health Organization, Fact sheet N°311, March 2011

Note to Reader

The knowledge I am sharing with you here has been part of my clinical work for some 40 years. In addition, I taught it to our soldiers when working with our military in Afghanistan. We human beings experience stress in peace and in war, and we can benefit from tools and training that help us to cope.

In this booklet you will acquire techniques that, through continued refinement and practise, have enabled many people to lead more effective, relaxed, productive lives.

The steps you are learning here are not difficult, though initially some may seem a bit awkward. Remember anything new may be awkward at first. But, you will find that with regular practise the steps will become second nature, reinforced by the benefit you'll find they bring into your daily life.

After you become familiar with and learn to apply the 5 Stress Relief Steps, you'll be in a very good position to tackle the challenge of weight control. Unlike most approaches to diet, I focus on **why** you eat. I assume you, like most people, know quite well what foods you should be eating, and what is not good for you. Chances are you are quite well 'diet educated', and likely had your share of trying this and that diet, losing weight, hitting a wall, or impasse, and then re-gaining weight you lost yet once again. The reality of so called yo-yo dieting has distressing familiarity for many.

My intention is to give you the knowledge and tools to help you avoid that.

Therefore, the first two parts of this booklet form two halves of a whole. Dealing better with stress will influence how you live your life, enabling you to be much more in control

Frank G. Sommers, MD

overall, including how, what, and especially why *you* eat. A recent Cochrane Library review[1] helps to illuminate the need to improve traditional lifestyle modification approaches to weight management.

Note: Please see the Resources section for informative advice on healthy nutrition. For those concerned with lowering cholesterol using dietary means please note the excellent research work of Dr. David Jenkins.

Stress and Food

As you well know, most of us (at least in North America) are not at our ideal or healthiest weight. In fact the term 'obesity epidemic' is appearing more and more frequently in the media, given that 500 million people across the world now are classified as obese. In North America, about half the adult population is overweight, with a third obese.

To check your personal weight/health condition, do the following. Determine your Body Mass Index (BMI), because this relates to Body Fat for most people:

Your weight in kilograms (kg) divided by the square of your height in meters (m) (Conversion: 2.2 lbs = 1 kg, 1 ft = 0.3 m) Example:

5'10" 190 lb person, that converts to 1.75 m, 86 kg

5 ft 10 in = [5 + (10 ÷ 12)] x 0.3 = 1.75 m

190 lb = 190 ÷ 2.2 = 86 kg

For a 5'10" 190 lb person, BMI is 86 divided by 3.06 (1.75 x 1.75) = 28 which is considered overweight. Over 30 would be obese. Healthy weight has a BMI between 18.5 and 24.9. This method applies to adults, over age 20, and is not an indicator of body fat in some people, such as athletes.

In addition to the BMI number, it helps to know your abdominal circumference, as weight around here tends to add to the dangers of being overweight. So take a flexible tape measure and wrap it all around at belly-button level: men should be under 40, and women less than 35 inches.

The excess weight most of us carry around impairs our mobility, impacts on our joints, heart, and blood pressure, and can damage our endocrine system, giving rise to alarming rates of diabetes, which in turn can have disastrous consequences on our health and longevity. Regrettably in 2008, globally, 374 million people were living with diabetes.

As you also know there is a huge 'diet industry' offering myriad remedies to help people shed weight. Occasionally, fads germinate and sweep our media, promising yet again a (usually) quick fix for the 'excess weight problem'. People, always hopeful, try this diet and that, in a wish for quick results.

However, the long-term story is often disappointing. The phenomenon of yo-yo dieting is well known to many who have tried, often with determination, to lose weight. Even when weight loss is achieved in the short term, the challenge of keeping weight off has eluded many.

What I call the 'stuck weight scale' phenomenon is familiar to most who conscientiously have adhered to a weight loss program. After a while you reach an impasse or plateau, even though keeping to your diet in a disciplined way.

As you may know, at this point your body is fighting, as it were, your attempt to lose more weight by adapting your metabolism.

The Body Weight Simulator is a new online tool (bwsimulator.niddk.nih.gov) to guide people in their weight loss quest in a scientific way. Dr. Hall's simulator will show us that we have to cut 10 calories per day for each pound of weight we want to lose. This means that for a 10 pound weight loss, you need to cut back 100 calories each day. And this must be permanent. You can expect half of this weight drop after one year, and almost all after three years.

To help you achieve this realistic goal, supported by science, my approach, as this booklet shows, deals differently with this serious personal and public health issue.

Here are some thoughts to 'chew' over:

- We rarely eat because we're truly hungry.
- Eating is a habit and a way of socializing.
- Usually we eat more than we need , especially when under stress.
- We eat foods we enjoy, and that make us feel good.
- But most importantly, food is our number one tranquilizer! Although often not recognized as such.

While some people have severe emotional eating binges, most of us turn to food (and some to drink) to comfort ourselves. We seek and can find temporary relief from painful feelings, such as anger, frustration, loneliness, sadness, and especially relief from stress. The term 'comfort food' is not a misnomer.

Informative new brain research[2] reveals how this might occur.

When a stress hormone floods the brain, it can temporarily rewire the part that controls feelings of hunger, or appetite. Thus a stress signal can be perceived as a hunger signal. The research also showed that eliminating the stress signal restored the ability to moderate the desire to eat.

Other brain research[3] found that obese people, when their blood sugar is low, have a stronger desire for high calorie food than average weight people. Again brain wiring may make it more difficult for obese folks to exercise willpower or food resistance.

Adding this reality to the inevitable stress in our lives, we see that brain wiring, or function, must be a key element in developing healthier ways of taking food and drink into our bodies. Thus we need to focus not only on when, what and how much we eat, but also, most importantly, **why** we eat.

The fast food industry found a niche by filling our bellies with yummy tasting, quick-to-consume food-items, (usually with a lot of fat, sugar and salt content) whose convenience, and time-saving features are very hard to resist. These are so-called 'obesogenic' foods.[4] That is, they promote obesity.

Further, in our culture, attractively packaged food is everywhere, available 24/7, as a salve for our emotional hunger or painful feelings, and we don't even need a doctor's prescription to indulge. Thus, in a way, food and drink have become the number one way we 'self-medicate'.

These realities inform the central strategy of my approach to overeating, and eating unhealthy foods.

We need to build resistance. This is a psychological quality, and I realize it can be a challenge to achieve. But the information in your hand now will make it easier, if you apply it. Allow this knowledge to be a gift to yourself. You deserve this life-changing 'food' for your mind.

I'm convinced that if we gain better control over stress in our daily lives, we'll be better able to improve our nutrition along with our physical and mental health, and thereby, the overall quality of our life.

Diets

I'm not a fan of diets of any kind. It is true that many diets can lead to weight loss, especially in the initial six months or so. However, reaching a plateau will discourage many who try dieting. Long-term maintenance of weight loss is also a challenge for those who have tried hard to lose excess weight.

The reality is that any excess calories we don't use up in our daily activities will find a home in our body as fat. Conversely, reduction of calories consumed will lead to weight loss, regardless of the kind of diet one follows.[5,6] But remember some diets can cause harm.

Moreover, weight gain can be a 'stealth' process. Research suggests that as little as 10 extra calories consumed per day can lead us to gain some 20 pounds in 30 years. Little wonder many of us first become aware of significant weight gain, when we put on our clothes, and find they don't fit right.

Important: Before embarking on any weight-loss program, it is always a good idea to get a medical check-up.

How to control your weight without dieting:

■ Take stock of how many calories a day you use up in your usual coming and going. For example:

Activity (1 hour)	Body weight 130 lb	Body weight 180 lb	Body weight 220 lb
Walking 2.5 mph	177 calories	245 calories	299 calories
Hiking, cross country	354 calories	490 calories	599 calories

■ Monitor the total number of calories that enter your mouth through everything you eat and drink per day. A small notepad in your pocket can help with this, as will the nutrition labels on the packaging, or information on the internet. Note, for instance, that a cup of Chocolate Mocha can fuel you with 580 calories, while a slice of Banana Loaf, or Apple Pie, or medium French Fries can be 400 to 500 calories!

■ **Remember:** Cutting back 250 calories per day (such as a small chocolate bar) leads to a weight loss of 25 lbs in 3 years, half of which should occur in the first year.[7]

■ Adjust your intake or output (e.g. work, activities, exercise) accordingly and remain realistic in your expectations. Be patient with yourself.

■ Keep in mind that the average person's daily need is:

Women:	2,000 calories
Men:	2,600 calories

Obviously, you'll need to be also increasingly choosy or mindful about the quality of food and drink you bring to your mouth. For example, remember that sugary drinks can be a significant addition to your daily caloric load.

A recent Harvard study documents the fact that some foods are bad for us (e.g. processed meats, French fries, potato chips), causing accelerated weight gain.[8]

A 2010 survey of consumers revealed that about half want healthier items on menus, but when dining out, only one quarter pay heed to nutritional values.

Maintaining your weight loss will depend on remaining mindful of what you eat and drink, and regular checks on body weight, along with being active or exercising.

But before you embark on this approach to managing your weight, you need to master ways to reduce and manage your stress, because stress so often leads to overeating.[9]

And this little booklet can help you do that.

Very Important: Complete your Personal Daily Weight Control Log. (See Appendix 3)

Do this honestly to the best of your ability long enough to give yourself a picture of how your food and drink intake vary with your activities, stress, sleep and mood. This simple tool can help you to make adjustments by increasing your awareness. You will come to realize that you are in control.

You will find that once you better control your stress with the tools you learn here, you will be more able to resist cravings triggered by negative emotions and stressful events.

So, give it a try. Put away those diet books and conquer your inner emotional hunger, and thus become able to powerfully resist the seductive foods and drinks that surround us. And if you occasionally yield to temptation, you'll still remain in control. And that is a good, worthy goal to adopt.

May this little work help you to achieve that.

By following my *5 Step Program* you will be in control, effectively managing your stress level, as well as your food and drink intake.

A new you is waiting to emerge.

My best wishes go to you on this exciting, life-enhancing, self-transforming journey.

References – Weight

1. Tuah NAA, Amiel C, Qureshi S, et al. Transtheoretical model for dietary and physical exercise modification in weight loss management for overweight and obese adults. *Cochrane Database of Systematic Reviews* (2011), 10:CD008066.

2. Crosby KM, Inoue W, Pittman QJ, Bains JS. Endocannabinoids gate state-dependent plasticity of synaptic inhibition in feeding circuits. *Neuron* (2011), 71(3):529-41.

3. Page KA, Seo D, Belfort-DeAguiar R, et al. Circulating glucose levels modulate neural control of desire for high-calorie foods in humans. *Journal of Clinical Investigation* (2011), 121(10):4161–4169.

4. Isganaitis E, Lustig RH. Fast food, central nervous system insulin resistance, and obesity. *Arteriosclerosis, Thrombosis, and Vascular Biology* (2005), 25:2451-2462.

5. Sacks FM, Bray GA, Carey VJ, et al. Comparison of weight-loss diets with different compositions of fat, protein, and carbohydrates. *New England Journal of Medicine* (2009), 360(9):859-73.

6. de Souza RJ, Bray GA, Carey VJ, et al. Effects of 4 weight-loss diets differing in fat, protein, and carbohydrate on fat mass, lean mass, visceral adipose tissue, and hepatic fat: results from the POUNDS LOST trial. *American Journal of Clinical Nutrition* (2012 Jan 18), [Epub ahead of print].

7. Hall KD, Sacks G, Chandramohan D, et al. Quantification of the effect of energy imbalance on bodyweight. *Lancet* (2011), 378:826–37.

8. Mozaffarian D, Hao T, Rimm EB, et al. Changes in Diet and Lifestyle and Long-Term Weight Gain in Women and Men. *New England Journal of Medicine* (2011), 364:2392-2404.

9. Ulrich-Lai YM, Christiansen AM, Ostrander MM, et al. Pleasurable behaviors reduce stress via brain reward pathways. *Proceedings of the National Academy of Sciences* (2010), 107(47), 20529-20534.

Resources

www.choosemyplate.gov – provides helpful information on how to eat a balanced diet.

ods.od.nih.gov – provides useful information on supplements

www.healthcanada.gc.ca/foodguide

www.eatrightontario.ca

bwsimulator.niddk.nih.gov – Body Weight Simulator

Cholesterol-lowering landmark diet study: an interview with David Jenkins, M.D. (http://findarticles.com/p/articles/mi_m0876/is_87/ai_n15338531/)

Jenkins DJ, Srichaikul K, Mirrahimi A, et al. Functional foods to increase the efficacy of diet in lowering serum cholesterol. *Canadian Journal of Cardiology* (2011), 27(4):397-400

Kong A, Beresford, Alfano C, et al. Self-Monitoring and Eating-Related Behaviors Are Associated with 12-Month Weight Loss in Postmenopausal Overweight-to-Obese Women. *Journal of the Academy of Nutrition and Dietetics* (2012), In Press.

STRESSRELIEF.drsommers.com

Those interested in Pathway Health Personal Weight Loss Coaching Program please contact: pathwayhealth@aol.com

PART III

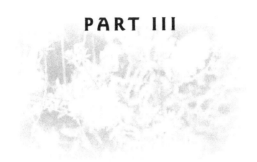

Make Better Love

Well, what about love?

In my experience we all need it. It's universal – even those who may proclaim "I don't". But, who really doesn't want, at least to be loved, even if they have difficulty giving love.

Thus, in my experience, working as a psychiatrist and medical sex therapist for close to 40 years, this issue of love is universally at our core as human beings.

To ignore this central reality of the human condition is to short change the millions of men and women whose love lives are not as fulfilling as they had hoped for, or indeed once was.

So, could emotional eating provide relief if you are hurt in love? Do you ever turn to food, and/or drink to give yourself comfort from the pain?

As I wrote in the section on WEIGHT, resilience, the ability to resist the ever present seduction of obesogenic foods is a critical tool in our ongoing battle of the bulge.

We also saw how stress can be converted by our brain into hunger signals. And 'love hurt' is surely stressful. As is all pain.

So once again we're back to dealing with our brain and stress circuitry. The re-assuring good news is, that the methods you learned in the section on STRESS, will assist you in a practical, effective way, to give yourself relief from 'love hurt' as well.

But there is more good news.

Over the years I have worked with thousands of men and women, singles, and couples some of whom were in quite good, satisfying relationships, where often everything in their life was fine, except in the bedroom. As a medical sex therapist I daily see folks who have difficulty making love. This can impose an enormous burden on the men or women so afflicted, and can also take a heavy toll on the relationship of a couple.

Here are some illustrative examples of this stressful reality afflicting single people.

———•·•———

This patient was referred following a suicide attempt on New Year's Eve for which he was hospitalized. He was a 27-year-old factory worker out for an evening of fun. He had attempted intercourse with a few women since age 18 and would lose his erection prior to penetration. He stated:

This New Year's Eve I spent in my friend's place. We had a few drinks and started to dance. As I danced with one of the ladies, I smelled her hair. I don't know why, but I got an erection. But this erection was much weaker than I remember years ago.

Frightened that he was going downhill sexually, and as he had tried to get help before with no positive results, he thought:

I don't know what I should live for. I know this problem is ruining my life. My life now is work eight hours a day, buy food, and watch TV. This is my daily program. On my day off I watch TV from morning 'till midnight. Is this life? I don't want to live all my life in a closed apartment and alone. I want to have girlfriends, maybe later a wife and kids. I am scared how I'm going to live the next 27 years. There can be a hundred people around, but I still feel alone with my problem. You can say "try to find a girlfriend," but no way. If I'm gonna find a girlfriend there is going to be a day when I have to have sex. What I'm gonna do then? I failed so many times I don't want to go over that again.

A 57-year-old school principal who lost his wife to cancer told me:

Nine months after my wife died I invited a lady out for dinner. She was someone I had worked with for seven years and a friend of my wife, although younger than both of us. (She was 41). I respect and like her very much, but found it difficult to get into the routine of asking someone out. However, having taken the initial step it was a very enjoyable evening.

We talked until three in the morning. I took her out several times. I don't recall exactly how many; but anyway, after a time we went to bed. I must admit I was rather surprised in that I did not expect that she would find me interesting in that our ages were fairly wide apart.

Things were going great in bed until we reached the point where she took hold of my penis for insertion and I ejaculated. My reaction and feeling at the time? Complete and utter devastation. I guess even humiliation; certainly failure. Here was someone I cared a great deal about, stimulated to a high pitch and disappointed. Since that time I have not on subsequent tries been able to get a full erection and have ejaculated. In this respect I guess it has gotten worse. How do I feel about the problem? It is the most debilitating thing I have ever tried to cope with. It has badly affected my self-confidence. It has made it difficult for me to communicate verbally with her. It is on my mind most of the time and affecting my concentration at work and my emotional stability – which I think has always been considerably high. Sometimes when by myself I simply break down and cry.

Now some examples of the couples I have treated:

Doug and Sandra are a hardworking couple in their late thirties. They met in high school and married shortly after Sandy turned 20. After two children, they immersed themselves in the usual preoccupation of young couples such as building a home, settling into jobs and looking after the children. Predictably, what was once a heated, spontaneous, romantic and exciting sexual life, abruptly went down the drain.

Sandy and Doug are not alone. There are thousands of couples like them. When they first met, both were quite emotionally, not to mention sexually, needy. Their happiness was complete in finding somebody they could really "talk to." The good sexual interaction – everything but intercourse – was a bonus.

By the time their second child was born, the couple was already headed for trouble. Doug was working late hours trying to establish himself in the business, and Sandy was trying to be a perfect wife and mother. Neither of them had any real sex education to speak of. So, when it came to addressing their intimate life together, it was really a situation of the blind leading the blind.

Doug had a rather strong sexual appetite. One of the things that he found so appealing in Sandy was her willingness to be flirtatious and sexually available. Eventually, however, they found themselves more and more in disagreement, especially over Doug's frustration about his unmet sexual needs.

Unfortunately, the more Doug pushed for sex, the more Sandy would resist. This started a vicious cycle of denial and physical frustration, and by the time treatment began, they reported that they had not made love for over a year. Their marriage was in crisis.

———•◆•———

John and Judy met 10 years ago, in their mid-20s, after being introduced by a mutual friend. They started dating and within a few weeks, their relationship blossomed into physical intimacy. Both were extremely content and happy – each feeling that they finally found "the one". Six months later, they moved in together and within two years they married with the approval of both their families. In their third year together, John and Judy decided to start a family and Judy promptly (on second try) became pregnant. However, despite their obvious happiness with one another, both noticed that in the period leading up to the pregnancy, while they remained friendly and enjoyed joint activities, their sexual interest in each other started to diminish. It was nowhere near as vibrant and energetic as it was in the first year of their relationship.

With the arrival of the baby, their sex life took an even steeper turn downhill. Blessed with a healthy young son, they were the consummate mother and father – they loved being parents. But more and more their affectional needs got pushed into the background, and neither paid too much attention, simply because they felt this was the way things were meant to be.

Two years later, their second child was born – not entirely planned, but neither unwelcome. However, the arrival of another baby reduced their sex life even more. Unfortunately, neither spouse urged counselling, and their sex life did not improve over the next six years they were together.

One year ago, Judy asked John to do something about his premature ejaculation. John was aware of this problem for some time and felt he'd been "coming too quickly" for the last four or five years. But since she had not complained about this, he thought all was well. By the time this couple came to see me, not only was their sexual desire for one another at an all-time low, but on top of everything else, Judy had hardly ever experienced an orgasm and certainly not in intercourse. History also revealed Judy was sexually experienced prior to meeting John, yet underplayed the importance of her pleasure. She generally saw men as pushy – wanting sex anytime, anywhere and as fast as possible – and accepted that this was how men were. Upon meeting John, she was taken by his gentle, easygoing manner, plus he made no demands on her sexually. "He seemed like a gentleman," she said. When asked if they feared their marriage was over, both John and Judy answered "yes".

———·•·———

Sarah and Sam have been married for seven years. Both come from different religious and cultural backgrounds – Sam is Caucasian; Sarah is Asian. They met, fell in love and eventually got married. Sam, who was used to more sexually assertive women, felt that with time, Sarah's sexual shyness would improve over the course of their marriage. But when Sarah gave birth to a baby boy, she devoted her full attention to being a mother. Sam appreciated Sarah's nurturing qualities, but felt that their sexual relationship was suffering badly. Their arguments increased as Sarah became more fatigued, as this usually happens, when taking care of a newborn and being confined to the home for most of the time. Sarah, eventually, rejected sex with Sam. As Sam's resentment grew, he turned to more solitary activities – watching TV or playing on his computer.

Both Sam's resentment and Sarah's rejection distanced the couple even further. By the time they came to me for therapy, the marriage was in serious difficulty as anger and resentment ruled their emotions.

———•—•———

Well, what about these very real life stories you just read. Often heart rending in their complexity, it's quite clear that each person is unhappy, and perhaps to different degrees, suffering.

I think you would agree that at some level they all were under stress. This would often be felt as being anxious or depressed.

Now, this is not the time or place to go into the details of how their treatment was done, nor their turbulent experience at times through it, but I'm pleased to say, they persisted and succeeded in turning their lives around. Some, on occasion have said at the end of therapy, "I feel a miracle has happened".

My work is very gratifying, especially when I hear comments like that, or receive notes of appreciation.

However, what I want to emphasize is that regardless of the particular difficulty in their intimate life, these, and all folks I treat, need to learn ways to modify their response or manner, in which they handle stress.

Stress is the psycho-physiological reality that is a common denominator in all these unhappy patients.

While clearly not everyone is suffering to the degree these people were when I first saw them, stress can and does have an impact on everyone's love life.

Thus, we come back to the title and subject of my little book.

As you have seen our ability to manage stress plays a central, crucial role in our ability to manage our life. As this ability improves we become stronger, more capable, empowered and resilient, better able to handle whatever inevitable curves life throws at us.

Thus we no longer need to feed our emotional hunger, or stressed out selves with unhealthy, obesity promoting foods that we know are not good for us.

As you become better able to treat yourself kindly and gently, you'll find your outlook on life will improve, along with your self esteem. You'll become a more positive, happier individual.

Indeed, a further benefit of this work may well be that your blood pressure, sugar, and cholesterol levels decrease, and your immune system strengthens.

In this little book I am sharing with you some of the knowledge and tools that over four decades as a doctor have been very helpful in turning around the lives of people, coming from all parts of our globe for help.

It has been a privilege for me to be part of their lives, and I offer you this little work in the spirit that led me to choose to become a healer so many years ago.

A note to those of you who may find this work challenging

I urge you to persist in your quest, and not give up the effort to find deep within yourself the loving and lovable person you were meant to be. Set yourself small, incremental goals, and use my **5 Step** program to help you with the ups and downs of your daily life. While your progress maybe slow, it will be rewarding, because by acquiring new life skills, you are becoming stronger, empowering yourself to live your life in a more fulfilling, happier way.

All my good wishes go to you on your exciting, life enhancing journey.

Resources

STRESSRELIEF.drsommers.com

goodsexnetwork.com

Enduring Desire: Your Guide to Lifelong Intimacy. Metz ME, McCarthy BW. Taylor and Francis, New York, 2011.

The Good Marriage: How and Why Love Lasts. Wallerstein JS, Blakeslee S. Warner Books, New York, 1996.

Frank G. Sommers, MD

Appendix 1:
Stress Immunization Wallet Card

This card maybe cut out, laminated, and carried in your wallet as a ready, helpful reminder of the '5 Steps'.

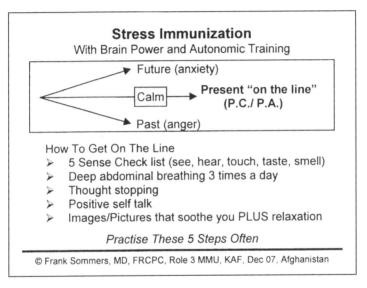

Figure 2

You may also download this information as an App from the **Apple Store** (Stress Relief by Dr. Frank) or **Google Play** (5 Easy Steps to Stress Relief). The enhanced download has a choice of soothing music and relaxing images, and a reminder feature.

See on the Web:
Stressrelief.drsommers.com
goodsexnetwork.com

or

Apple Store:
Stress Relief by Dr. Frank

For Android Mobiles (Google Play):
5 Easy Steps to Stress Relief

Appendix 2:
Relaxation Images

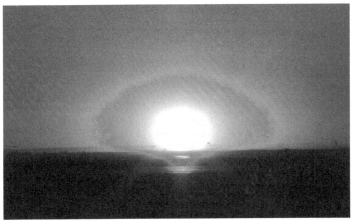

Frank Sommers

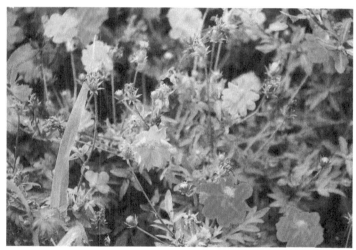

Frank Sommers

Frank G. Sommers, MD

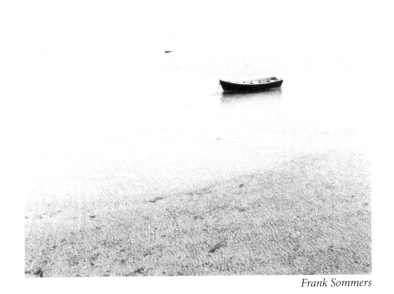

Frank Sommers

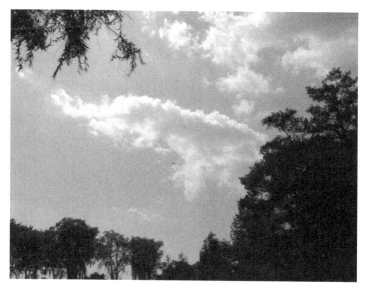

Frank Sommers

Frank G. Sommers, MD

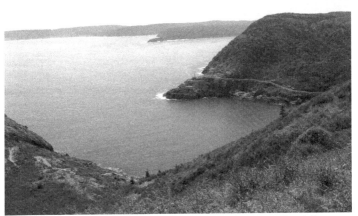

Frank Sommers

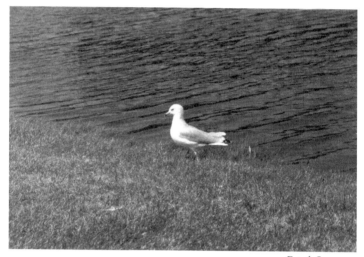

Frank Sommers

Frank G. Sommers, MD

Appendix 3:
Personal Daily Weight Control Log

Date: _____

Day: Mon / Tues / Wed / Thurs / Fri / Sat / Sun

Current Weight:_____   Blood Pressure:_____

Target Weight: _____   Cholesterol:_____

	Food Eaten & Drinks Consumed	Qty	Cals	Fats
Breakfast				
Morning Snack				
Lunch				
Afternoon Snack				
Dinner				
Evening/ Night Snack				
Total				

Physical Activity (min.):_____

Sleep (hrs):_____

Overall Stress: Low / Medium / High

Mood: Low / Negative / Positive / Variable

Copyright © 2012 Frank G. Sommers, MD

Date: _____

Day: Mon / Tues / Wed / Thurs / Fri / Sat / Sun

Current Weight:_____   Blood Pressure:_____

Target Weight: _____   Cholesterol:_____

	Food Eaten & Drinks Consumed	Qty	Cals	Fats
Breakfast				
Morning Snack				
Lunch				
Afternoon Snack				
Dinner				
Evening/ Night Snack				
Total				

Physical Activity (min.):_____

Sleep (hrs):_____

Overall Stress: Low / Medium / High

Mood: Low / Negative / Positive / Variable

Date: _____

Day: Mon / Tues / Wed / Thurs / Fri / Sat / Sun

Current Weight:_____   Blood Pressure:_____

Target Weight: _____   Cholesterol:_____

	Food Eaten & Drinks Consumed	Qty	Cals	Fats
Breakfast				
Morning Snack				
Lunch				
Afternoon Snack				
Dinner				
Evening/ Night Snack				
Total				

Physical Activity (min.):_____

Sleep (hrs):_____

Overall Stress: Low / Medium / High

Mood: Low / Negative / Positive / Variable

Date: _____

Day: Mon / Tues / Wed / Thurs / Fri / Sat / Sun

Current Weight:_____   Blood Pressure:_____

Target Weight: _____   Cholesterol:_____

	Food Eaten & Drinks Consumed	Qty	Cals	Fats
Breakfast				
Morning Snack				
Lunch				
Afternoon Snack				
Dinner				
Evening/ Night Snack				
Total				

Physical Activity (min.):_____

Sleep (hrs):_____

Overall Stress: Low / Medium / High

Mood: Low / Negative / Positive / Variable

Frank G. Sommers, MD

Date: _____

Day: Mon / Tues / Wed / Thurs / Fri / Sat / Sun

Current Weight:_____   Blood Pressure:_____

Target Weight: _____   Cholesterol:_____

	Food Eaten & Drinks Consumed	Qty	Cals	Fats
Breakfast				
Morning Snack				
Lunch				
Afternoon Snack				
Dinner				
Evening/ Night Snack				
Total				

Physical Activity (min.):_____

Sleep (hrs):_____

Overall Stress: Low / Medium / High

Mood: Low / Negative / Positive / Variable

Date: _____

Day: Mon / Tues / Wed / Thurs / Fri / Sat / Sun

Current Weight:_____   Blood Pressure:_____

Target Weight: _____   Cholesterol:_____

	Food Eaten & Drinks Consumed	Qty	Cals	Fats
Breakfast				
Morning Snack				
Lunch				
Afternoon Snack				
Dinner				
Evening/ Night Snack				
Total				

Physical Activity (min.):_____

Sleep (hrs):_____

Overall Stress: Low / Medium / High

Mood: Low / Negative / Positive / Variable

Frank G. Sommers, MD

Date: _____

Day: Mon / Tues / Wed / Thurs / Fri / Sat / Sun

Current Weight:_____   Blood Pressure:_____

Target Weight: _____   Cholesterol:_____

	Food Eaten & Drinks Consumed	Qty	Cals	Fats
Breakfast				
Morning Snack				
Lunch				
Afternoon Snack				
Dinner				
Evening/ Night Snack				
Total				

Physical Activity (min.):_____

Sleep (hrs):_____

Overall Stress: Low / Medium / High

Mood: Low / Negative / Positive / Variable

Frank G. Sommers, MD

Those interested in personal training or coaching please contact Pathway Health at:

Email: pathwayhealth@aol.com

Phone: 416-922-4506

Fax: 416-922-7512

Presentation of Dr. Frank Sommers '*Stress Immunization by Training Your Brain in 5 Easy Steps*' Program can be arranged. Please contact pathwayhealth@aol.com

CPSIA information can be obtained at www.ICGtesting.com
Printed in the USA
LVOW011304201212

312571LV00005B/5/P